TICKED OFF

TICKED OFF

A Physician Shares How He Beat Lyme and Got His Life Back

Dr. Gordon Crozier

TICKED OFF

Copyright © 2018 by Dr. Gordon Crozier

Published By:
Utmost Press
70 Main Street, Suite 23-MEC
Warrenton, VA 20186
www.UtmostPress.com

Print ISBN: 978-0-578-41530-7

The Origin of My Work in the Treatment of Lyme Disease

*I*n the early 1970's, a relatively small cluster of children who regularly lived and played in heavily wooded areas of Lyme, Connecticut, began to experience inexplicable symptoms of sudden fever, joint pain, and debilitating neurological disorders. While the range of symptoms did appear to be unprecedented, they did in certain respects mimic similar symptoms of chronic fatigue syndrome, fibromyalgia, rheumatoid arthritis, and in some cases, even mental illness (*including depression, anxiety, and ADD*). The symptoms gradually began to subside and even resolve in some children, while others continued to experience debilitating and even lifelong health problems. Similar symptoms also appeared in other children throughout New England and the upper Midwest, even going back into the 1960's. In every single case, it was later determined, the afflicted child had been bitten by a tick prior to the onset of the mysterious illness.

I was one of those children.

At the tender age of eight, my entire young life was flipped upside down after I was bitten while playing in the woods in northern Minnesota. I very quickly transformed from a fun and adventurous little boy into a sickly, bed ridden, and depressed invalid. A host of pediatricians could make no sense of my poor health and, of course, not a one of them ever thought to ask my mother about any potentially dangerous insect bites. Although my childhood symptoms eventually subsided, they would go on to reoccur throughout my teenage years and then well into adulthood.

Suffice to say, I was never the same after my 8-year-old experience with a chronic, mysterious ailment that each and every doctor seemed completely unable to properly diagnose or adequately treat. I never once received anything like a proper diagnosis and not even once did any doctor inquire regarding insect bites. For years it remained a miserable mystery which completely confounded every physician or specialist my parents and I would so desperately reach out to for help.

My chronic illness, however, did provide the singular motivation which propelled me to study and practice medicine, which I still practice today as a Board-Certified physician near Orlando, Florida. During my many years of practice, I was privileged to deliver babies as an OB/GYN, to research and practice neurology, and also to have the opportunity to instruct resident physicians at the University level. But--*due directly to the painful circumstances of my own health*--I also managed to carve out time for countless hours spent researching the root cause of my *own* condition, which still plagued me, while focusing all of my medical experience on finding the cause of my ongoing illness, and then hopefully discovering *the cure!*

I eventually shifted my focus into the areas of alternative, genetic-based, and integrative medicine, because my more "traditional" medical colleagues, and my "standard" research methods had, up to that point, offered me no clear-cut diagnosis, no reliable answers, and absolutely no real hope.

Because I myself have experienced chronic illness, I've always been able to tap into a well of deep compassion for my patients. And while many doctors may avoid seeing or dealing with the complications of patients with chronic, seemingly inexplicable symptoms, because of my own condition, I've always understood my responsibility to welcome my fellow sufferers with open arms. Quite a few years ago one of my patients complained to me about remarkably similar symptoms to my own, which included: *intermittent chronic pain, muscle weakness, occasional flu-like symptoms, and nonspecific anxiety and depression.*

Of course, I was easily able to feel deep compassion for her suffering because I knew *exactly how she felt!* In fact, I was--*unfortunately for my profession*--the first and only doctor to believe her. Together we went on to explore multiple aspects of her symptoms, as well as their sudden onset, when on one visit she almost inadvertently happened to mention to me that she'd been bitten by a tick just prior to the onset.

A tick bite! I will never forget that moment.

Could it be possible that a tiny insect bite might be the cause of my patient's illness (as well as my own)?

To make our long story short…our answer was- YES!

I'll dive into greater detail in the following pages, but the following days, weeks, months, *and years* would turn out to become both exhilarating and maddening. I was excited to have finally found my diagnosis--*and hopefully my cure*--but also angry because traditional medicine had so completely failed us both. I became almost obsessed with the countless numbers of sufferers out there who remained continually sick and frustrated just as my patient and myself had been for so long. In short, I was *TICKED OFF*, and so I began to devote all of my time and my practice to the emerging, effective treatment of Lyme Disease.

I began to research Lyme Disease *exclusively*; reading about it, consulting with other physicians, medical researchers and scientists, and then working directly with hundreds of patients who all expressed similar symptoms.

What I quickly discovered is that some of my patients remembered being bitten by a tick, while many others did not. Yet they all had the same symptomatology!

I also studied the DNA of all my Lyme patients, something no other doctor in the world was doing at the time. I took DNA samples from every patient and then randomly compared them to each other, attempting to get at the ROOT CAUSE of their disease on a cellular level. What I discovered through my DNA research and analysis helped me develop customized treatment plans for *each individual Lyme patient*, based on their *unique DNA structure*.

Eventually Lyme patients began to visit my practice from all over the world, from France, Australia, Canada, even Africa. Once again, I was able to directly connect with the compassion I felt for all my Lyme patients because not only did I sympathize with their pain and suffering, I also understood their frustration!

Some of my patients eventually found complete and total remission, while others were able to much more effectively manage their disease. Yet all of my fellow sufferers were completely and gratefully freed from that frustration as together we learned how to clearly recognize and effectively minimize their symptoms.

When I began researching and treating Lyme Disease, little did I know that incidents of Lyme would soon accelerate to epidemic proportions. In the early days it was quite rare for a Lyme patient to find me. But today Federal Government data recently showed that *10 times as many people are contracting Lyme* as are diagnosed with Type 1 Diabetes! Lyme will soon become the polio, mumps, and measles epidemics of our generation.

In the interest of full disclosure, I must allow that I haven't *completely* cured my own Lyme Disease as of yet, and I may well live with some symptoms the rest of my life. But I *do* feel like a new man today with an energy and vitality that surprises even my own family.

I no longer live in fear, frustration or anger regarding my symptoms, having completely conquered the great majority of them, and *effectively managed all of them*.

I feel better today than I've felt in 50 years. Like so many of my patients, Lyme had consumed too much of my life for far too long, and it's been an incredible feeling of freedom to finally break free of its chains.

In these short pages I want to share with my fellow sufferers what I've learned about Lyme, and what I've learned about how to treat this manageable malady. Of course at this point in my career I'm certain I could write an entire textbook on Lyme, having treated so many patients, but my purpose here is to give you a perspective on Lyme you almost certainly have never heard before. I continue to spend many hours working with my patients towards their unique solutions, so I've learned a lot from them during their journey toward health and healing, as well as my own.

I want to share some of that journey with you on these pages.

I want to share with you:

- **The Crucial Importance of a Proper Diagnosis**
- **The Many Signs and Symptoms of Lyme Disease (and how to recognize them as such)**
- **How Knowledge and Understanding of Your Unique Genetics (your DNA) Can and Will Help You Find Relief (and even a cure)**
- **10 Things You Can Do NOW to Alleviate Your Lyme Symptoms**
- **How Certain Patients Can Find Faster and Longer-lasting Remission Using IV-Therapy.**

The current medical facts regarding **Lyme diagnosis** are these-

Almost all doctors today use the Western blot test-- exclusively--*to diagnose Lyme.*

What my years of research and practical treatment have proven to me, however, is that while the Western blot test can *sometimes* confirm the presence of certain antibodies to accurately diagnose Lyme *(similar to an HIV diagnosis),* the existing and continuing problem is that *the Western blot fails to diagnose Lyme in the majority of patients, the majority of the time!*

And for a number of reasons which I'll explore at greater length in the following chapter.

As a direct result of this disturbingly common misdiagnosis, however, *more than half of my patients test negative for Lyme with Western blot. (including those who actually remember being bitten by a tick)*

Just imagine if 50% of patients (or more) *were misdiagnosed with diabetes, HIV or cancer?*

This is nothing short of a medical catastrophe!

Through my research and work with hundreds of patients, I've developed a protocol which accurately diagnoses Lyme Disease in roughly 70% of those patients who previously tested negative for Lyme with the Western blot.

So how do my tests result in a more accurate Lyme diagnosis?

The science is fairly straightforward.

Lyme Disease is a strain of the *Borrelia burgdorferi* bacteria left behind in the body after a tick bite. The *Borrelia burgdorferi* can cause, in some people, certain antibodies to naturally develop in order to fight off the bacteria. The problem for Lyme sufferers is that some people (*most patients*) never develop these antibodies, or, their natural supply of antibodies developed then dissipated from the body before or after the testing. Lyme, therefore, is *not* like HIV in this way, as a similar antibody test for HIV is nearly 100% accurate. Sadly, for myself and my fellow sufferers, too many doctors these days take the easy path to diagnosis and treatment of Lyme (*the exclusive use of the Western blot test*). I discovered that during my battle with my own health. But, now, when I get on my knees and pray at night I thank God for my Lyme. Why?

My disease *compelled* me to take the harder road that lead to a far more accurate and far more reliable diagnosis.

Occasionally, some of my colleagues tell me that what I do in treating Lyme is revolutionary, but I don't think so. I think it's just good old-fashioned medicine. I got "ticked off" and I didn't give up. That's the way every good doctor should always progress towards proper diagnosis!

Why is it So Difficult to Test for Lyme Disease?

Regarding the accurate diagnosis of Lyme Disease, we can gain insight on the long and very difficult road for healthcare practitioners focusing on this disease. These challenges are not only educational, but also involve successfully overcoming the idea that Lyme does not exist in certain geographical locations. The reality is that *Lyme exists everywhere*. With a quick internet search, you can currently and easily find at least eight different medical associations specifically focused on the diagnosis and treatment of Lyme disease. These various associations, however, collaborate very rarely and some, *not at all!* As in all politics, each has their own agenda, with each maintaining different ideas and practices regarding the treatment of Lyme disease.

As of this writing, almost all diagnostic tests currently available for detection and confirmation of Lyme have a widely variable sensitivity and test specificity, **depending to a very great degree on the stage of infection.** It's this most difficult aspect of accurately identifying and verifying the presence of Lyme that makes its correct confirmation very difficult. In light of this, we can understand more clearly that it's crucially important for all medical professionals to monitor the literature on available testing for Lyme, and then to utilize--*and promote*--those tests which perform most effectively and most directly address the concerns of the afflicted patient.

With over 300,000 new cases of Lyme Disease diagnosed each year, it's difficult for me to believe that so many physicians either ignore or outright reject the possibility of Lyme in so many patients. However, diligent practitioners who take their time to properly identify *Borrelia burgdorferi*, become suddenly and evidently aware of the dangerous effects of Lyme. Some medical professionals still refer to Lyme as the "Great Masquerade," because its symptoms mimic many other diseases. With over 100,000 estimated patients seeking medical care for Lyme symptoms that could not be properly diagnosed, far too many patients were treated for these symptoms, and never properly treated for Lyme. As a commonly misunderstood disease, Lyme is severely under diagnosed, and therefore often goes untreated.

I do not believe in treating only symptoms. Instead, we must look and find the root cause. We must be proactive so that our patients can have legitimate hope that we can reliably diagnose their symptoms before treatment.

However, many healthcare pro-fessionals remain unaware of accurate, available, FDA approved tests (*beyond the Western blot*) like ELISA and ELFA tests, or how these tests can help in their diagnosis. I personally don't blame healthcare professionals entirely as regrettably, there is still inadequate education and a good deal of misinformation in this field of medical study. It can also be difficult to conduct testing depending on the particular facility's resources, and the insurance paperwork involved is often daunting for clerical staff. In addition, many of these tests (*including immunoblot tests like Western blot, immunosorbent tests like ELISA, or fluorescent immunoassay tests like ELFA*) are seldom covered completely by insurance companies—*which will lead to critical gaps in an accurate diagnosis*--and therefore will not be recommended by certain physicians participating in HMOs. As an unfortunate example, it's far too common for physicians in Georgia, Alabama and Florida (*as well as other states*) to incorrectly inform patients that Lyme Disease (*and the specific type of tick which carries Lyme*) does not even exist there. I believe this gives patients a false sense of security, despite their own certainty on the likelihood of Lyme Disease.

Do these physicians even read articles which indicate other sources for Lyme? I don't know, but I *do* know that after finishing their residency, due to time constraints, the vast majority of physicians read very few medical articles outside of their own particular specialty.

So, how can we know where Lyme Disease is going to be more prevalent in upcoming years? Looking at the data, the areas in the United States where Lyme disease will expand and/or explode in the next few years certainly include the states above, in addition to many others. Many veterinarians are proactive in testing dogs, and other animals, for tick borne illnesses. Because of this, we know Lyme is spreading in these states, and other areas with potential Lyme infestations. We also know that ***according to the CDC, Lyme has been diagnosed in every state***, and variants of *Borrelia burgdorferi* has been found around the world. Though many countries have only one of over 30 different species of *borrelia*, the threat of Lyme still exists worldwide, as well as in our own United States, making it all the more crucial that we should take the unchecked spread of this disease seriously, and make every effort to deal with it comprehensively.

The European country of France, for example, is very proactive about identifying and alerting their citizenry to their Lyme specific forests. They don't try to specifically differentiate between differing types of tick species, however, because they realize more than one specific form of tick carries borrelia. Throughout the heavily forested areas of their nation, the French healthcare authorities prominently display signs demonstrating how to properly remove ticks, as well as how to prevent ticks from latching onto your skin. It is amazing to me that France is so proactive in warning its citizens as to the dangers of Lyme, and I am personally thankful that they're so aggressive in Lyme Disease prevention. As a direct result of their proactive efforts, France now has only 30,000 Lyme diagnosis' annually, while the US suffers from over 300,000.

I find it quite interesting that the French have been so proactive in the prevention of Lyme Disease as we can clearly see that Lyme Disease is not just an American problem. There are now also over 15 reliable research articles stating that ticks are not the only vector in transmitting *Borrelia burgdorferi* to humans. This is not only invaluable information on our understanding of Lyme, but also a major issue moving forward.

A New Hope for Accurate Lyme Disease Testing and Diagnosis

Up to this point I hope that I've stressed the absolutely essential need for reliable testing for Lyme, as this is the critically important first step in the accurate diagnosis and subsequent treatment of this disease. Another of the ongoing difficulties in accurately testing for Lyme, however, is that *all* of the current testing methods of immunoblot (*like Western blot*), immunosorbent (*ELISA/enzyme-linked immunosorbent assay*), and fluorescent immunoassay tests (*ELFA/enzyme-linked fluorescent immunoassay*), each have strengths that are helpful and dependable in detection, but each also has critical blind spots which can often lead even a diligent general practitioner—*who may not be especially well versed in the detection of Lyme-*-down the wrong path in terms of their diagnosis. Up until now, a two-step combination of these tests (*EX: an ELFA test followed by the Western blot*) is generally regarded as the most accurate method to verify and confirm the presence of Lyme but, of course, this two-step process is time consuming as well as a burden on many insurance plans.

Quite often, inadequate insurance plans will fail to cover one or the other in the vital two-step process, thus leaving the patient completely exposed to a misdiagnosis which could have been avoided.

The gap in accurate detection occurs when or if the two-step process is bypassed (*due to insurance restrictions or physician neglect based on misinformation*), and/or when the Western blot test is bypassed for any number of reasons the patient has little to no control over. This is a critical mistake in the fact that *all* Lyme Disease testing measures a patient's antibody (or immune response) to the borrelia bacteria which cause Lyme, but both ELISA and ELFA tests are designed to be extremely sensitive; meaning that when they're used properly, almost everyone with Lyme Disease will test positive, and this is good news in terms of detection. The bad news—*and crucial detection difficulty*--is that it's also possible to test positive with *an ELISA/ELFA* test even when you do not have Lyme Disease. This *false positive* frequently occurs because of a host of other common medical conditions (including *Epstein-Barr, bacterial endocarditis, lupus, certain gum diseases, et al)*, hence the necessity of the Western blot/two-step verification method. This complex testing process, of course, also explains why so many physicians may be reticent in employing the ELISA/ELFA tests, as a false positive is an unfortunately common outcome, which may not be necessarily successful in detecting the presence of Lyme.

The great news in terms of accurate detection, however, is the cutting-edge emergence of *chemiluminescence-based antibody testing* specifically designed to more accurately detect and verify the presence of Lyme in patients who have already been treated with commonly prescribed antibiotics. Our office has vigorously pursued the use of *chemiluminescence* as the most advanced and accurate method of testing, especially in the very common cases of patients who have visited us after other medical measures (*prescribed by other medical facilities*) have completely failed to alleviate their symptoms. Chemiluminescence testing has proven to be critically important in these cases, as so very often our new—*and still suffering*—patients have already started down a course of antibiotic regimens prescribed by their previous physicians. The ongoing problem with the presence of common antibiotics, as regards the detection of Lyme, is that *all patients in the early stages (initial 30 days)*, **especially those previously treated with antibiotics, may not exhibit detectable levels of antibody** *(immune response)* **using only the standard testing methods of ELISA/ELFA, which in turn can lead to false negatives.** This of course can lead to further misdiagnosis, further treatment mistakes, and further suffering for the frustrated patient.

The promise of chemiluminescence is that this test *(which employs a special, chemically reactive light that is 2x times more accurate than standard ELFA, and up to 4-6x times more accurate the chromogenic-reactive ELISA)*, in our experience, has put a reliable end to the false negatives that occur with most ELISA/ELFA testing. This is especially important in the very, very common cases of patients who have been frustrated in their inability to receive an accurate diagnosis for their continually deteriorating health, despite their numerous visits to a range of medical facilities and doctor's offices.

Another strength of chemilumi-nescence testing is that, in sharp contrast to ELFA/ELISA/Western blotting systems, chemiluminescent antibody detection takes place when energy from a chemical reaction is released in the form of light. The most popular chemiluminescent substances are luminol-based (*ELISA tests are not*). During this process, in the most layman's terms, luminol oxidizes and forms an "excited state product" which emits light during testing as it decays to its "ground state." This type of light emission occurs only during the enzyme-chemiluminescent substance reaction, making the chemiluminescence method far more sensitive, and significantly more accurate. The further significance of the chemiluminescent test is that it is not prone to the false positive reactions, as a result of other non-Lyme conditions, due to its unique chemically produced effects. It is these types of false positives in standard ELISA/ELFA tests that, as mentioned previously, can so often lead even the most thorough physician down the wrong diagnostic path.

Chemiluminescence testing has proven to be a reliably accurate method for us and we always strongly urge all our patients--*especially those patients who have sought previous help but found little to no relief*—to take advantage of this technology. As doctors and caregivers, I do feel it's our responsibility to find answers for patients who have found none so far. As a person who has struggled with Lyme for great portions of my own life, I fully understand and appreciate how vitally important it is to finally find the relief that has been sought for so long, and to finally have an answer to the universally frustrating question of- *What else can I do now?*

There *is* real hope for those Lyme sufferers who have not yet found their specific answer, and it is up to us as physicians to position ourselves in the ideal place to offer that hope.

Our National Addiction to Prescription Medications

Considering the significant amount of time your average medical facility spends on the administrative demands of medical records and medical coding--*rather than direct patient care*—it's no wonder modern American medicine is falling behind other advanced nations in its diagnosis and treatment of Lyme disease. As physicians, I understand that we must advocate for patients *ourselves*, as well as for the future of our own medical protocols. While many physicians will select the type of continuing medical education and financial support offered by "Big Pharma," most of this type of strictly prescription-based information and education focuses on the treatment of symptoms *only*. Of course, this is all a symptom itself of our own modern All-American, quick fix, instant gratification culture today.

Sure, we all want the convenient solution of simply taking a pill to make our symptoms instantly disappear but instead, we would be better serving ourselves if we all refocused on searching for the root cause of our conditions so that we can find reliable, long-term solutions which are much healthier for us in the long run.

As I write this, and to my great dismay, *approximately 60% of the American population takes more than one prescription medication every day!* At one point, when I was a clinical faculty member, we took the time and effort to review comprehensive, nationally compiled medical statistics which revealed that the average state resident patient was typically prescribed *at least five types of medication per doctor's visit.* Even children!

Clearly, this would be a strong indication that too many of our medical professional ranks are moving in a direction that is not necessarily based on the best medical practices as they relate to a patient's overall health and long-term wellbeing.

When we combine this flood of "Big Pharma" marketing and distribution success with the billion-dollar "nutraceutical" industry, both the number and frequency of potentially harmful prescription drug interactions is astoundingly frightening. While it's difficult to estimate the total number of fatalities due to unnecessary prescription interactions, reliable estimates from the last two decades show that over 100,000 deaths occur each year, due directly to prescription medication overdoses, and/or prescription interactions. Indeed, an article published in the 1998 *Journal of American Medical Association* stated that 106,000 deaths were projected to occur as a secondary result of medication interactions or complications.

In addition to this distressing news, we should all understand that even herbs and other "all-natural" supplements can negatively interact when used in addition to prescription medications. Some herbal "all-natural" medications can certainly be dangerous, such as the interaction between popular *Serotonin Uptake Inhibitors (commonly prescribed to treat depression/anxiety)* and *5-HTP* which can result in an unhealthy and potentially dangerous serotonin surge. In far too many cases, lack of specific information regarding how different herbs or supplements interact with prescription medications can cause detrimental, dangerous effects, or even result in fatalities which could have been avoided. I have had numerous patients visit with a prior diagnosis of a chronic disease/condition, only to discover after reviewing their prescription medications and supplements regimens that they had been taking substances with the clear potential of dangerous interactions. By simply taking my patients off of these types of entirely unnecessary drug combinations, many improved both dramatically and immediately with no further treatment.

I have also personally seen the devastation that unnecessary drug interactions can cause, firsthand. Years ago, my father accidentally suffered a minor fall, and subsequent intracerebral bleeding occurred, bleeding which was easily treatable and, once treated, would have been manageable for my Father. As a physician, I also knew that this bleeding was due directly to the fact he was on a blood-thinning medication as a result of a cardiac valve replacement as a child, following a traumatic fever.

After being admitted to the hospital, correctly evaluated, and then properly treated following his relatively minor adult accident, the hospital staff thought it best that he be placed in a physical rehab program before coming home. When he arrived at the rehab center, however, the staff there *failed to read his medications list properly,* and so he was administered another patient's prescription medication (*which happened to be for Parkinson's*) before any staff—*or myself*--was able to detect the mistake. Disoriented and unable to stand on his feet as a result of the side effects from the unnecessary drug combination interaction, my father fell again, this time suffering far more serious injuries to his face and upper torso.

While the facility initially denied ever giving my father any improper medication, upon my arrival following the second fall and after an immediate review of his chart, I knew what had happened and was appalled that apparently, certain healthcare professionals are far more concerned with protecting themselves from medical liability than they are with the actual care and wellbeing of their patients! The terrible ending for my father, and his loving family, was that he was never able to fully recover from that second—*and entirely unnecessary*--fall, and so he spent his final years needlessly bouncing from hospital to care facility until he finally passed away. This was one of the most difficult lessons I ever had to learn concerning the state of our medical community and the prevalence of prescription medication and its very serious potential for misuse. I trust that it is a lesson we can all learn from, and learn to avoid by paying the strictest attention we can to our use of all prescription medications.

When it comes to the prevalence of prescription medications, however, the FDA is not always the "bad guy." The federal Food and Drug Administration *is* there to help protect our citizens and our society, and in general can be relied on to carry out their duties with professionalism and critical scientific scrutiny. Our present healthcare reality however-- *considering recent, decade long trends*—is that we must acknowledge that the FDA may be at least as complicit in the widespread proliferation of prescription medications as the manufacturers of Big Pharma. I do find this alarming as the FDA *should* be working hard to help find the best treatment modalities for every disease and disease system, in spite of the big pockets of private industry that may or may not control certain areas of opportunity that come with an ability to bankroll their products to the front of the approval line. Often, government agencies forget that they are put in power by *We the People*. As physicians, however, we must continue to work together with the FDA, the CDC, and our state-run medical agencies in order to establish the best, most reliable, affordable and effective treatment for every patient we encounter, properly and legally.

Lyme Disease Symptoms and How to Reliably Identify Them

Let's take a closer look at some signs and symptoms of Lyme disease, and why so many patients—*and doctors*--may miss this critical diagnosis. As I previously noted, Lyme carries with it a wide range of symptoms common to many conditions, and the devastating effects of Lyme Disease may also include: *fatigue, night sweats, cognitive impairment, Alzheimer's, dementia, psychosis, depression, mood swings, fibromyalgia, other neurological presentations, rheumatoid arthritis, MS, Parkinson's, and ALS.* Unfortunately for we sufferers of this difficult to diagnose condition, these are

only an incomplete list of possible symptoms—
and a frustratingly diverse one at that-- which may
indicate the presence of Lyme. Let's drill down
into some of the specifics that may allow a better
understanding of potential symptoms, a better
list of questions you may want to ask yourself,
and as a result, a more accurate diagnosis should
you have to visit your doctor.

The "Bull's Eye" Rash (and other methods of transmission)

Most individuals who contract Lyme
Disease either *do not* or *cannot recall* ever being
bitten. And even in the rare cases when they
do recall a bite, many *never directly relate* what is
commonly referred to as a ***"Bull's Eye"*** rash,
to that tick bite. In another frustratingly difficult
to diagnose aspect of this condition, this "Bull's
Eye" rash (*a distinct bullseye-shaped redness on the
surface of the skin which may expand up to 12"/30cm*)
commonly presents itself anywhere between 3
- 30 days *after* the initial bite. This widespread
time lapse makes it all the more difficult for the
patient to easily or precisely connect the initial

tick bite to the distinct rash itself, or to the onset of symptoms that *will* follow and then, of course, to report that crucial information in any clear manner to their physician upon initial visit when the symptoms present (*almost always after a further delay associated with the slow onset of symptoms*). It is, therefore, much too common for this rash to be treated as an insect infection, or skin affliction entirely unrelated to Lyme, especially in areas of the United States where Lyme disease is not commonly thought to exist. In addition to the difficulties of identifying and reporting the initial rash, many studies suggest that only 20% of those who contract Lyme will, in fact, ever even develop the "Bull's Eye" rash.

In my practical experience, however, that number has been closer to 4-6%, *with over 90% of patients showing no rash at all*. I may add, I have also seen the distinct "Bull's Eye" rash develop from bites that were not tick related in any manner. This can be and is a real issue, as Lyme is primarily known to be a tick borne illness. Though it is not well understood and at present there is no medical consensus--*and may even be ignored by the greater medical community*--there are several reliable Lyme research studies which demonstrate that mosquitoes can, in fact, carry Lyme Disease as well.

Of course it is not my desire or my purpose as a medical professional to start or promote any hysterical frenzy by stating that there are other carriers of Lyme Disease, but given my professional experience, I do feel that we must be rational and understand the possibility of mosquito-borne Lyme may exist. With a number of medical associations, like the *Lyme Disease Association of Australia*, pinpointing articles regarding the transmission of Lyme by more than just ticks, we must be proactive in seeking the ultimate answer. In recent years more and more research studies and published articles are finding that mosquitoes, fleas, mites, and other sources are possible causes of Lyme Disease. A German study also reported a case of a fly transmitting Lyme Disease, resulting in arthritic changes. French studies have also stated that mosquitoes are a possible carrier for B*orrelia* (*Lyme Disease*).

I myself once treated a previously healthy young teenage girl who had been involved in a motor vehicle accident. She had required several blood transfusions as a result of her injuries, yet despite a full recovery from the injuries resulting from the accident, she was never able to achieve lasting health and wellness again, and suffered from a range of debilitating symptoms relating to a chronic condition her family doctor had been unable to diagnose or, of course, effectively treat. Unfortunately, as I had never treated her prior to her accident or subsequent transfusion, I was unable to ever definitively prove what the precise circumstances of her chronic condition may have been, but I did and do believe she contracted Lyme Disease from the transfusion.

The possibility is always in the back of my mind, and so it is my plea to those *fellow sufferers who have been accurately diagnosed with Lyme Disease to avoid giving blood if it is at all possible.* Although in many cases, donating blood is a commendable act of charity, in the case of my fellow Lyme sufferers, it may be best if we can express our charitable efforts in different areas. Even more worrying for potential donors who may have Lyme and not know it or may have been improperly diagnosed, on most occasions the bacterial infection has already dug its way through and clear of the circulatory system, rendering blood tests inaccurate.

Certain studies have even indicated that Lyme can be sexually transmitted, and therefore on some spectrums should be considered an STD.

And what about our national blood supply?

Do blood donation/collection facilities frequently test blood for Lyme?

Getting accurate information regar-ding these questions is difficult even for those of us in the medical professions but, I think it is information we must continue to seek nonetheless. I think of it frequently when I see the blood donation vehicles outside of movie theaters, urging people to donate. Make no mistake- *We all need these critically important donations.* But what if we're transmitting Lyme Disease through that very same blood? I know for most, this is a scary thought, but in my professional experience, I believe we must endeavor to move forward into further research regarding this possibility, and then create an effective medical strategy/prevention program.

Bell's Palsy

Bell's Palsy is a serious Lyme-related condition (*commonly resulting in slight to severe paralysis to one side of your facial muscular system*) which I personally, and very unfortunately, experienced in my teenage years. Once while traveling with my High School team band, I was quite embarrassed to discover a significant droop to the left side of my face--*which my bandmates had either very politely or uncomfortably ignored*--all while performing in front of a crowd! It wasn't until we had a performance break and my then best friend directed me to a mirror that I discovered, to my horror, the condition of my facial muscles and understood that my symptoms had once again presented in a most embarrassing form. It was another of the painful lessons regarding Lyme that has always stuck with me.

Because the causes are commonly due to a range of conditions, it can often be diagnosed general that this serious form of facial paralysis also (incomplete sentence)

When researching all possible causes of Bell's Palsy, one will first see the causes commonly listed as-

1. *Unknown*
2. *Viral infection*
3. *Possible inflammation due to unknown causes.*

Yet to date, many medical professionals have a limited understanding regarding the more recent medical literature showing the causes and indications for this condition.

I have personally treated many patients with Bell's Palsy who were previously instructed by other doctors, *"not to worry, it's a self-limiting problem, and will likely go away with time…"*.

Now in many cases, including my own, this unfortunately embarrassing but usually temporary symptom/condition does recede on its own. However, I have also seen cases of individual patients who were left with permanent facial paralysis as a result of Bell's Palsy left unchecked. If we can find the root cause of this condition, perhaps we could also degrade, impede, block or entirely halt the initial onset of Bell's Palsy as a result of Lyme Disease. An early detection of symptoms here may also help prevent other adverse neurological effects inflicted by the onset of Lyme.

General Fatigue

Fatigue is of course an extremely common malady, and an all too common symptom for a wide range of conditions, which also happens to affect more than 76% of individuals with Lyme Disease. It is, however, very difficult to find a root cause for this debilitating symptom, as it also presents as a result of a multitude of possible everyday origins. One of the first things a physician or practitioner will look at to treat fatigue is, of course, the particular patient's daily workload. Of course if a patient's stress or daily workload is too high, this may in many cases, merely indicate that the overworked, stressed out patient—*which accurately describes far too many of us*—simply needs a break! The other most common aspect typically examined in regard to fatigue, and especially chronic fatigue, is the patient's *viral load*.

In just one example, many individuals have contracted the common infection of *mononucleosis (mono)* in the past, which typically produces elevated viral loads unrelated to Lyme, but continued elevated viral loads of the *Epstein-Barr* virus can also be an indicator of chronic fatigue. In fact, 99% of Lyme patients I have treated have also had elevated levels of *Epstein-Barr*, entirely unrelated to any history of *mono*. This correlation has led me to theorize that perhaps there is a deeper connection between *E-B* and Lyme Disease.

Fatigue, however, is an extremely elusive symptom, and is rarely taken seriously enough by one's family members, family practitioners, or even the patients themselves. Most individuals just don't know how to properly address, or what to do when it comes to chronic unrelenting fatigue. For example, a patient of mine with unrelenting chronic fatigue went to several general practitioners with no positive results. She then visited *integrative doctors*, as well as *functional medical doctors*, who performed a large workup specifically designed for adrenal fatigue. Her cortisol levels and the rest of her workup were all subsequently determined to be normal. She was subsequently treated for *Epstein-Barr* with no results and her condition then continued to further decline.

Finally, she came to me and I was able to run a test which came back positive for *Borrelia Burgdorferi - Lyme Disease*.

And so, after numerous, frustrating visits to numerous facilities, together we began the long process of pulling these harmful biological toxins from her body, and her fatigue began to slowly resolve as she gradually regained her health, along with her youthful vigor.

Fibromyalgia

Fibromyalgia is very often associated with chronic fatigue, and both conditions commonly may happen to present almost simultaneously, making it even more difficult to differentiate the root cause of either, and to properly diagnose this cause in any effective treatment for both. The biggest difference between the two, however, is that fibromyalgia typically includes significant widespread pain, due to overactive, overworked nerve endings. This condition causes significant muscle pain, nerve pain and insomnia, as well as the ever-elusive symptom of fatigue. Perhaps the true cause of fibromyalgia may be Lyme Disease, though the majority of cases I have seen suggest to me that overexposure to mold may be the main underlying culprit of fibromyalgia.

Night Sweats

Night sweats are another common symptom of Lyme Disease. However, night sweats are also another case of a difficult to pin down symptom which can be related to any number of factors, conditions or disease processes as well (*such as tuberculosis*). Therefore, although night sweat symptoms may be related or connected to Lyme Disease, we must *first rule out all the other possible disease processes* in order to make an accurate Lyme diagnosis. This elimination process is of course, a drawn-out system of undoubtedly painful trial and error, but one any responsible physician must not ignore.

Cognitive Impairment

Cognitive impairment is a common complaint of Lyme patients, due to *neuroborreliosis*, a neurological manifes-tation of Lyme Disease. *Neuroborreliosis* impairs neurotransmitters, receptor sites, and releases *endo* and *exo*toxins, resulting in a significant, disturbing mental decline that may present is a number of ways that can include: *confusion, memory loss, loss of balance and even vision impairment.*

Depression and Psychological Problems

Psychological changes are a common effect of *neuroborreliosis* as well. In a published journal of psychiatry, over 30% of the psychiatric patients studied showed signs of *Borrelia burgdorferi* infections which resulted in *neuroborreliosis*. The very promising news, however, is that many patients accurately diagnosed with, and then accurately targeting Lyme disease in their treatment have completely reversed their neuropsychiatric behaviors.

I have experienced the onset of these symptoms with patients in my office as well. Some psychiatric disorders common in Lyme patients can include: *memory impairment, dyslexia, seizures, anxiety, panic disorders and attacks, psychosis, violent behavior, rage, mood swings, sleep disorders, ADD/ADHD, and obsessive-compulsive disorders*, in addition to the number one most common psychiatric disorder- depression.

I once treated a wonderful patient who visited our clinic, a vibrant youngster we'll call "Sam." Sam was an active, social child who loved playing basketball and was always an eager student in school. Prior to his visit with us, however, he very suddenly and inexplicably found that he was losing his ability to read at the level he had already achieved. Then he began to lose his ability to read altogether and his horrified parents quickly brought him to us for help with this terrifying condition. My heart went out to Sam, because like him, I too at one time had found myself in the same situation as a child. His story was my story.

When his symptoms and his reading disability first presented, his confused parents at first did not know where to turn as several weeks went by, and then Sam's symptoms worsened. He began to experience inexplicable exhaustion—*seemingly unrelated to his level of physical activity*--and could no longer participate in basketball or any of the activities he previously enjoyed. His parents noticed the gradually disturbing change, as Sam grew reclusive and was no longer his normally talkative self. In response over the following months they took him to numerous physicians, psychiatrists and psychologists, but to no avail. By this point Sam had begun to hear voices, and had completely withdrawn from his normal social structure and school activities. Diagnosed with severe depression and possible schizophrenia, he had visited over 22 physicians and been placed on several medications to combat his auditory hallucinations.

After those terrible months of confusion for his family, Sam's mother tearfully informed me that he was just a shell of who he once was, and told me that I was their last hope. His parents just wanted their vibrant young boy back.

It was difficult to examine Sam. He appeared fearful, would not speak and expressed convulsive alarm at any physical contact. After our tests were finally completed, we had our diagnosis - Lyme Disease, *Bartonella*, and *Ehrlichia*. He started receiving a treatment regimen designed to specifically target this diagnosis and symptom after symptom after symptom began to resolve. It was a slow, painful process, but Sam was improving.

Eventually, on a day I will never forget, I noted a once again bright-eyed, playful, active Sam and his grateful father tossing a football together outside my office window just before their visit. As I write this, Sam has just graduated high school at the top of his class. In light of my own struggles with this condition, and witnessing firsthand its terrible impact on Sam's wonderful family, the pure joy of seeing this young man once again actively rejoining and happily contributing to his own welfare and the advancement of all his worthy goals, is one of the greatest gifts it has ever been my genuine pleasure to receive as a physician.

Arthritis

Arthritis was one of the first symptoms noted among the children in Lyme, Connecticut-- *the town for which Lyme Disease was unfortunately named*— and remains one of the more common symptoms of this condition. Arthritic pains related to Lyme can be extremely intense, and as a consequence of their severity, patients are often misdiagnosed with *rheumatoid arthritis*. When performing an aspiration on the joints of many affected arthritic patients, *spirochetes* are commonly noted, a potentially Lyme-related bacteria. If practitioners are not specifically looking for Lyme, however, a simple misdiagnosis of rheumatoid arthritis will completely miss the underlying causative agent, resulting in a treatment regimen that is moving in the wrong direction until it can hopefully be set right.

ALS / Lou Gehrig's Disease

I would like to take a moment to tell you of a young mother who visited my office with a diagnosis of ALS. At the time of her first visit, "Martha" was in a wheelchair and appeared beaten and hopeless, her voice was extremely weak, and she seemed to be at the end of her rope in terms of her health prospects. Despite her condition and without prompting, once in my office and with her very fragile voice, she immediately informed me that she could get out of the wheelchair for the exam, if needed. I was deeply touched by her strength through all her adversity, and my entire staff felt deep compassion for Martha, and then quickly fell in love with her gentle, peaceful, yet quietly determined ways.

After presenting her with the truth of a correct diagnosis--*that Martha had tested positive for borrelia burgdorferi and mycotoxins*--we began her properly aligned treatment for her Lyme. Due to the severity of her ALS, it was a slow process. During the initial treatment her weakness accelerated, but after some time I noticed she was able to step out of her wheelchair to walk more and more easily. I also began to note that with each passing visit she was speaking more clearly and forcefully. Even her family had begun to notice and was excited about the clarity of her speech and her newfound energy. Upon one of her last initial treatment visits, she was speaking very clearly, and walking without even the use of a cane!

In short, Martha had hope again. She truly was getting better. We repeated her Lyme numbers, which were completely gone, and her mycotoxin levels, which were again normal. After we completed her initial treatment, she then returned for a three month follow-up. Martha told me of how, glowing with excitement at her progress, she had met with her own neurologist. After glancing at her chart, he said nothing and walked out of the consultation room. Poor Martha had no idea if her visit was complete, but she was promptly informed by the nurse that she would not require another visit there. Her treatment with us had made further treatment with her own specialist unnecessary. I am not ashamed to admit that as Martha continued to progress, our office regularly threw parties in honor of her courage and commitment.

Although not everyone with ALS has Lyme Disease, over 50% of patients I have treated for ALS tested positive for *borrelia* recurrence. Patients we treated for Lyme Disease often returned to their standard medical facilities and family doctors with their symptoms greatly improved. I've even heard from our patients of unfortunate cases in which general practitioners-- *upon witnessing drastic improvements in patients that had previously shown little to none*--simply allowed that these patients must have been misdiagnosed due to administrative or "patient error." Rather than enthusiasm for the strenuous recovery, these practitioners instead appeared astonished, aggrieved and occasionally resentful that they had not been the medical expert who had effected the positive course of treatment. Of course I find it extremely distressing in instances like this, however many or few, in which the medical community cannot work together as a whole in a positive and educational environment committed to patient health and wellbeing as the common, and solitary goal.

As physicians, we all take an oath. That oath orders us- "First, do no harm." Although it's not always considered as part and parcel of our oath, this commitment to healthcare translates to *emotional harm* as well as physiological. When we physicians truly care for our patients, we should be nothing more or less than purely excited for them when they are able to achieve health and wellness, regardless of the particular circumstances of their treatment. We all want every single patient who walks out of our practice to have hope, a happy life, and a future filled with health and wellness.

We physicians should always strive to "work ourselves out of a job." If or when we are unable to do so, we're simply hanging on to every patient in an atmosphere more focused on business than health, and so moving in the wrong direction.

Autoimmune Disorders

The exact causes of autoimmune diseases are still poorly understood and require further, deeper research. At present what we *do* know is that autoimmunity is a response in which our own body quite literally "attacks" itself. Like rheumatoid arthritis, there are several autoimmune diseases which have been reliably associated with Lyme Disease. For instance, it is estimated that approximately 45% of those with Lyme have *Hashimoto's thyroiditis* as well (*the most common cause of hypothyroidism in the US*).

We typically see individuals with specific genetic SNPs (*single nucleotide polymorphisms indicating genetic variation between individuals based on a single DNA building block sample*) which can be related to specific types of autoimmune disease, such as a genetic predisposition to *lupus, thyroid conditions*, or *Crohn's disease*. While not every individual with autoimmune illnesses have Lyme, it may be worth further investigation in order to find as yet undiscovered connections. Knowing an individual's genetics can help practitioners understand certain genetic predispositions, and then investigate the possibility that biotoxins may activate these genetic SNPs. For instance, research thus far indicates that some individuals with the markers for P53, HLA-DR4, TNF alpha, IL-1, (*and other genes*) may be predisposed to certain types of autoimmune diseases. Although it is not yet clear, scientific research seems to point towards a genetic aspect, combined with other additional elements, which can push specific genetic expressions. These other elements may include diet, lifestyle, environmental toxins, and biotoxins.

I know I may differ from many other physicians in my belief, but my experience demonstrates that it is crucial to combine all aspects of modern medicine to see the totality of an individual, and thus to provide the greatest, most reliable treatments specifically geared directly towards individual body health and wellness.

A former patient, who was previously treated with eight different high-dose antibiotics for extended periods of time, once visited my office to address her chronic health problems. I immediately saw that Lyme seemed to be tearing her body apart, causing increasing arthritic changes to the point of near deformity. Due to the *spirochetes* completely destroying her joints, she had been scheduled for a joint replacement and had come to me to confirm her diagnosis before she underwent the major, life-changing surgery. Her surgeon, to his credit and informed by all his experience, had instructed her that he would not perform the surgery until her joints had definitively tested negative for *borrelia*. After examining her, we were able to ascertain that long-term, high-dose regimens of antibiotics had totally destroyed her digestive process. Her normal *gut flora* was completely gone, and as a result, she was having a hard time eating any normal food at all, and had been suffering from an extremely limited and improperly nutritious diet. Worst of all, her previous physicians had failed to realize that the *borrelia* had quickly become resistant to the antibiotics. Indeed, a great deal of reliable research indicates that *borrelia* becomes resistant within 72 hours of being exposed to specific antibiotics. Over the next several weeks, we continued to work with her, and finally were able to clear her joints so she could return for surgery.

Antibiotics are of course an indispensable tool of proper medical care in countless instances, but in regards to Lyme and autoimmune diseases, I believe that we need to do more research on exactly how long it takes for *spirochetes* to become resistant to treatment, and which antibiotics are truly the best option for specific patients with specific conditions.

My Conclusions Concerning Lyme Disease and its Treatment

I am forever thankful for the patients and physicians who have been given a chance to share their stories and struggles with this elusive disease which I've personally dedicated a great deal of my career towards. I am thankful too, for celebrities and other well-known personalities who have publicly shared their own struggles with Lyme Disease. Recent news of the role stem cell treatment has added to the list of tools in the recovery from Lyme is more and more encouraging with each passing day. We need this type of advanced research, and we need to remain proactive throughout our entire medical community. Far too many Lyme patients have hit rock bottom, and so are entirely dependent on friends and family to pull them back to the light of life. Those patients without proper family support, in too many cases, can't even afford most treatments due to insurance restrictions. While there are alternative methods of getting approval, these are extremely expensive, as practitioners must follow the guidelines the FDA has set forth in governing proper medical treatments.

Way back in the 1960's of my youth, physicians did not bill your insurance for you. They simply, clearly and honestly provided the service, gave you all the information you required, and then you presented the bill to your insurance company. I believe if we still did things that "old-fashioned" way, we would see a revolt from patients who would be forced to continually fight to force their insurance providers to pay for their very necessary procedures. I know that battle. When individuals are paying a monthly premium ranging from $1,800 to $3,000, I find it extremely difficult to maintain my own patience with insurance companies that refuse to pay for their "clients" in desperate need of medical care.

The present political world of medicine is as frightening to me as I suspect it is to the average citizen looking for proper healthcare for themselves and their families.

- How is this helping Lyme patients?
- Why have doctors given up control?
- Why do patients just submit?

I believe that certain healthcare policies have taken a giant step backwards in terms of the overall health needs of the average patient, and so call upon individuals to take back control of their health. Practitioners - *We must take control of our position once again as well.*

I am, once again, "ticked off" because we have sat silently and idly by while others are dictating to us what kind of treatment modalities we will provide for our patients. This is flat wrong. As physicians, we must fight too, and we must fight for our patients.

For many of us healthcare professionals treating Lyme Disease, we have sometimes put our license on the line - *especially in a few slow to scientifically evolve states.* I believe if we could work together on a united front, even when we choose to treat Lyme disease with differing methods, we could all make a difference. I often wonder where we would be today if there was a more united medical professional front to help push Lyme Disease to the top of the scientific research priority list. If we had such a united effort to pursue these goals, perhaps we could encourage new, and necessary, treatment modalities. These new studies could then not only benefit our patients, but eventually drive healthcare costs down to a more fiscally responsible level.

It seems that now all of medicine has become a protocol scheme. Now protocols have their place, but I believe in treating the individual. And most individuals just don't fit protocols. In fact, most of my patients have failed every protocol known to man! I have seen patients on blood pressure medications with no history of elevated blood pressure. They had been placed on the medication due to hospital protocol, and if they were not given this specific medication the hospital would be penalized and would or could not then receive full payment for services rendered. I think this is a ridiculous waste of invaluable resources, as well as deeply detrimental to public health.

In our society, we may need to submit ourselves to protocols at this time. However, individuals with specific genetic expressions may not fit existing protocols well, if at all. Some patients may display specific symptoms, even though the cause for these symptoms are significantly different from a patient with similar symptoms in the very next bed.

Should both patients receive the same protocol? I don't believe they should.

This is food for thought, as we explore our options, and then perhaps push back against the current, restrictive insurance industry "nepotism" controlling our medical society.

As a physician, and a patient, I believe we should have hope. Hope is what we must cling to when our greatest gift of health fails us. Without it, we have despair; and that despair will fill every cell in our bodies until we can hope again. Without hope, we will not respond optimally to treatments, and so cannot be at our healthiest. Even today, more and more physicians and practitioners are looking outside of the box, as traditional medicine has left them with no answers, no patience, and no hope.

> *"Hope deferred makes the heart sick, but a dream fullfilled is a tree of life."*
> Proverbs 13:12

This scripture comes to my mind frequently And though I would never wish to give false hope to my patients, I know that hope is something we all must find for ourselves nevertheless. Therefore, I have hope, hope and God Almighty. He is our Defender, He is our Healer, He is our everything. Cling to Hope.

Dr. Gordon Crozier

Crozier Clinic

1301 South International Parkway
Suite 1041, Lake Mary, FL 32746
www.CrozierClinic.com
407-732-7668

CPSIA information can be obtained
at www.ICGtesting.com
Printed in the USA
LVHW052003160919
631220LV00007B/1355/P